Healing

A Woman's Guide
To Recovery After
Mastectomy

Rosalind Dolores Benedet, N.P., M.S.N.

R. Benedet Publishing
San Francisco

Library of Congress 93-90627
ISBN 0-9637917-0-2

Illustrations by Shannon Abbey
Edited by Edith A. Folb, Ph.D.
Production Coordination by M.J. Coleman
Cover Design by Curium Design
Typesetting by Bonnie Monohan

R. Benedet, Publishing
220 Montgomery St., Penthouse Suite
San Francisco, California 94104

 printed on recycled paper

This book is dedicated in memory of Judy Diane Hill
1947–1991

Thanks

The thoughts and efforts of many people have gone into this book. I sincerely appreciate each person's contribution.

Shannon Abbey

Mellownee Bassett

Derrick Bowyer

Pattie Bryson

Susan Claymon

Ferris Crane

Richard Cohen, M.D.

M.J. Coleman

Susan Diamond, L.C.S.W.

Loren EsKenazi, M.D.

Edith Folb

Roberta DeFrancesco

Phillip Gordon, M.D.

Diana Karlsen

Patricia Lazowska

Pamela Lewis, M.D.

Estella Liu

Sharron Long

Linda T. Miller, P.T.

Bonnie Monohan

Roni Peskin Mentzer

Ricki Pollycove, M.D.

Ralph Roan, M.D.

David Ronce

Peter Richards, M.D.

Michael Small, M.D.

Theresa Sommerville

Evan Sornstein

Joy Sornstein

A special thank you to:

M.J. Coleman

Edith Folb

Sharron Long

Contents

Healing

A Woman's Guide
To Recovery After
Mastectomy

1.
About This Guide

This guide is designed to aid your physical and emotional healing. Though you will have the support and care of a team of health professionals, you are truly the most important person on your health care team. A positive attitude, open patient-doctor relationships, and realistic information about what lies ahead will give you the tools to speed your recovery.

This guide offers practical and easy-to-understand information on what to do on a day-to-day basis. Knowing what to expect and how to take care of yourself should lessen many of your concerns and allow you to actively participate in your treatment plan and recovery.

Your doctors, nurses, and other members of your health care team are your best source of information about your care and recovery. The information in this guide will add to their advice.

We hope this guide will contribute to your recovery and healing.

2.

Before Your Surgery

Talking With Your Doctor

In the weeks and months to come, you'll probably have a number of questions and concerns about your recovery. You are encouraged to bring all your questions and concerns to your doctors. The unknown can be very scary, but information about what lies ahead can reduce some of the anxiety that you may have. Being informed about your treatment plan will allow you to play an active role in your recovery.

As we've said, you are key to your recovery. A strong desire to recover, along with other positive feelings — love, determination, faith, and humor — go a long way towards your healing. As important is developing an open relationship with your doctors. This largely depends on your ability to speak frankly with your doctors. They need to know what you're thinking and feeling so that they can prescribe the best treatment and resources for you. They also need to know how much or how little information you want from them.

Write down your questions and concerns as you think of them and bring that list with you to your visits. Remember, there is no such thing as a "silly" or "dumb" question.

Sometimes it's difficult to remember discussions with your doctors. You may find it helpful to take notes and/or ask a friend along to help you remember what is said. Also, you can ask your doctor if you can tape your conversation.

Don't be shy about asking the same questions over again. It's not always easy to take in all that the doctor is saying. Simple statements like, "I know that I asked this before, but I couldn't remember all that you said," or "Can we talk about it again?" help both you and your doctor to focus on important information.

Ask your doctors about the best method for talking to them about your concerns. By telephone? At a special appointment? At a regular visit, with more time scheduled in for discussion?

Remember you are the best judge of your own body — don't ever be embarrassed to bring your concerns to the attention of your health care providers.

Immediate Breast Reconstruction

Since you are about to have breast surgery you should be aware of breast reconstruction as an option. Although it is gaining popularity, many women are still unaware of it. Reconstruction may be done at the time of the mastectomy (immediate reconstruction) or at any time after the surgery.

A mastectomy with immediate breast reconstruction is a surgical procedure in which the breast is removed and the breast contour is rebuilt. An advantage of immediate reconstruction is that you need undergo only one general anesthesia and one period of hospitalization rather than two.

There are several types of reconstructive surgery. These include using an implant behind the chest muscle, or taking tissue from your belly, back, or buttocks to rebuild the breast contour. The nipple and areola may be rebuilt at the same time or later on. Several factors are taken into account when deciding about reconstruction, such as the type and stage of your tumor, your weight and whether or not you smoke.

If you are interested in immediate reconstruction, ask your surgeon for a referral to a plastic surgeon. You will need to consult with the plastic surgeon before your mastectomy. Immediate reconstruction requires that your surgeon and the plastic surgeon coordinate the surgeries.

Breast reconstruction is not for every woman. Even if you think you may want reconstruction, you may not be ready to make that decision before your mastectomy. Remember, there is no pressure to decide before surgery. Breast reconstruction can be done at a later time.

Informed Consent

Before surgery, you will be asked to read and sign a consent form. Signing the form means that you have been told about the procedure and its potential risks. It also means that you understand your surgical options and agree to have the recommended surgery performed. You should be given the form in advance of your surgery, so you can look it over and raise any questions or concerns with your surgeon. Some of the questions you might want to ask your surgeon are:

◆ What kind of procedure are you recommending?

◆ What are the risks and side effects of the procedure?

◆ Am I a candidate for immediate breast reconstruction?

◆ Am I a candidate for a lumpectomy (a procedure that removes the cancer and preserves the breast)?

◆ What are the advantages and disadvantages of one treatment over another?

◆ How long will I be in the hospital?

◆ How should I expect to look after the operation?

Your Stay in the Hospital

We suggest you pack lightly, since your stay in the hospital will be a short one. Usually, you will be discharged in one to three days after your surgery. Most hospitals will provide for your personal needs (i.e., tooth-paste, soap, body lotion, comb). If you prefer, bring your own favorite grooming products (i.e., face wash, face cream, etc.). Since all your jewelry, including rings, earrings and such will be removed before surgery, you may decide to leave these at home.

When packing, think about bringing along some special clothing that will make it easier for you to dress after surgery. Some suggested items are:

◆ A loose-fitting blouse, shirt or dress that buttons in the front. It will be more comfortable for you to put on than a pull-on garment or one that buttons or zips in the back.

◆ A soft tee-shirt or camisole. This will be much more comfortable than a bra after your surgery.

PADDING

Some women prefer to go home without padding after surgery; others drape an attractive scarf over their chest. For those who desire it, a lightweight, temporary breast form can be worn home from the hospital. You can make your own temporary breast form by using a foam rubber or cloth covered shoulder pad. Whether a shoulder pad or some other form, the material used should be soft and lightweight. You can safety-pin this temporary breast form to the inside or outside of your undergarment. More will be said about these forms — both temporary and permanent — in the section on breast forms on page 45.

3.

The Day Of Surgery

*H*ospital procedures differ. You may be admitted to the hospital the day before your surgery for routine tests, such as blood tests and chest x-ray. Most likely, you will have these tests done one or two days before surgery, and be admitted to the hospital the morning of the surgery.

When it's time for your surgery, you will be asked to undress completely and put on a hospital gown. Your jewelry, wallet and other personal items will be taken and placed in a secure place; these will be returned to you after surgery. If you wear dentures, a hearing aid, contact lenses or glasses, they also will be safely put away and brought to your hospital room after your surgery. Just before your surgery, you may be given some medication to help you relax.

Then, you will be taken to the operating room on a gurney (a bed with wheels), in a wheelchair, or you may be asked to walk accompanied by a nurse. Before you are put to sleep, an intravenous line (IV) will be put into your arm to provide you with necessary medications and fluids. The surgery will take between two and four hours, depending on the procedure.

When you wake up in the operating room, one of the first sensations you may notice is that you are cold. You will be covered with a warm blanket. From the operating room, you will be brought to the recovery room. In the recovery room, a nurse will frequently check your temperature, pulse, blood pressure and chest bandage. The nurse also will make sure you are comfortable and will give you medication for pain or nausea if needed.

You will spend about an hour or two in the recovery room before being brought to your own hospital room and settled into your bed. Most women continue to feel drowsy during these first few hours after surgery. If you feel pain or nausea, you will be given medication.

When you're fully awake, you will be encouraged to sit up in bed, take deep breaths, and cough. This helps clear out your lungs and prevents any potential lung complications. About four to six hours after your surgery, you will be asked to get up from bed and walk. The first few times, your nurse will help you.

You'll be given clear liquids, such as Jello, clear broth, and tea, four to six hours after surgery. Your IV will be removed, as soon as you begin drinking liquids and as long as your temperature is normal and no medications need to be given by IV.

Having Visitors

Although visitors are not allowed in the recovery room, you may have people come see you as soon as you are settled in your own hospital room. But, you may not feel like having visitors or even telephone calls right away. This is perfectly okay. Family and friends certainly will understand.

Preparing for Discharge from the Hospital

You will be discharged in one to three days after surgery. Before you're released from the hospital, your surgeon will come by to examine you, review discharge instructions with you, prescribe pain medication, and arrange a follow-up visit. Finally, your nurse will go over the discharge instructions with you one last time.

4.

Your Recovery At Home

Many women say they feel surprisingly well the second day after surgery. Even so, if you experience pain or discomfort, take prescribed medication as needed. Many women will resist taking pain medication because they worry about becoming dependent on it. Remember that pain medication is generally needed only for a few days and nights, so dependency is not really an issue. Being comfortable allows you to be physically active and to get your needed rest. Both are important for healing and recovery.

You may notice that you have less energy than you normally do. Don't be discouraged; slowly, your energy will increase. You may also notice that your arm and chest are temporarily swollen from the surgery. To help reduce swelling, rest your arm comfortably on several pillows so that your arm is resting higher than your heart. In addition, perform the "Arm Pumps" exercise demonstrated on page 24. Do this about three times a day.

Bed rest is not encouraged because inactivity and bed rest tend to lead to more fatigue. We recommend that you stay physically active.

However, some women do benefit from a nap during the day. A good rule of thumb is to "do what you feel capable of doing." A few guidelines for appropriate levels of activity:

◆ Use your affected arm. Gentle motions are recommended. (See page 23 for more information on arm exercises.)

◆ Allow family and friends to help you with housework and the preparation of meals. If you want, you may do some moderate housework, such as preparing a simple meal or washing a few dishes. Avoid strenuous lifting, pushing or pulling, particularly with your affected arm.

Looking at Your Incision

The first time you look at your incision in the mirror can be a difficult moment. Some women prefer to be alone the first time. Other women find it comforting to be with someone they trust, such as their spouse, partner, friend or surgeon. Some women want to see the incision right away, right after surgery; others put off looking at their incision for a few weeks. There is no right way or right time. You must do whatever feels best for you. However, it is important that you do look at yourself in the mirror so that you can begin to feel comfortable with your new body.

If you are having difficulty looking at yourself in the mirror, try looking down at your incision. Some women find that looking down at themselves, rather than looking in the mirror, is easier on them emotionally. Whatever way you choose to do it, looking is important to make sure your incision is healing properly.

You may notice bruising and swelling in the chest and underarm area. The bruising and swelling are temporary and will slowly disappear. Although an infection at the site of the incision is unlikely, you should observe it for signs of increased redness, drainage, swelling, warmth or pain. If any of these conditions develop, call your surgeon.

Your incision may be closed with either metal staples or steri-strips (a special type of tape). If you have staples, your surgeon will remove them at your first follow-up visit. If you have steri-strips over the incision, they will fall off by themselves about 10 days after surgery. If the steri-strips get wet, just pat them dry.

Caring for Your Incision and Drain

Although taking care of your incision may sound intimidating, it's really a straightforward and easily managed process. When you are discharged, you may have a dressing over your incision. If so, just keep the dressing dry. The incision won't heal properly if the dressing stays wet. Your surgeon will remove the dressing at your follow-up visit, about five days after your surgery. Sometimes the dressing is removed before you go home from the hospital.

TAKING CARE OF YOUR DRAIN

*I*f you don't have a drain, you can skip this section. If you're not sure if you have one or not, ask your surgeon or hospital nurse.

Drains may be inconvenient and not very pretty to look at, but they 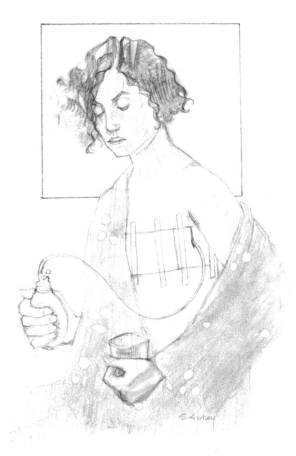 serve a necessary function. They may be placed under the skin during surgery to remove blood and fluids that collect as part of the healing process. You may have one or two drains in place. If so, they may be removed before you are discharged from the hospital. It is more likely, however, that you will go home with your drain in place.

If you do go home with the drain in place, you will need to empty it.

INSTRUCTIONS FOR EMPTYING YOUR DRAIN

*E*mptying your own drain is easy. Your nurse will review the following instructions with you before your discharge from the hospital:

1. Wash your hands.

2. Remove the plug from the pouring spout and pour the contents out.

3. Measure the contents. A measuring cup may be used.

4. Flatten the drainage container and replace the plug into the spout.

5. Record the date, time and amount of drainage. (See page 88 for "Drain Care Chart".)

6. Empty the container two times a day (i.e., when you get up in the morning, and before going to sleep at night).

7. Look at the skin around the drain. If you notice increased redness, swelling, warmth, pus or pain, call your surgeon.

8. Safety-pin your drain to your blouse or underclothes. Always keep your drain below the level of your armpit.

As you heal you will notice that you will have less drainage, and the color of the drainage will change from red to light pink to a light, straw-colored yellow.

Instructions for Changing Your Drain Dressing

You may have a drain dressing. If you do, then change the drain dressing just once a day, or whenever it gets wet. Before your discharge, your nurse will go over the following steps:

1. Wash your hands.

2. Remove the old dressing and throw it away.

3. Look at the skin around the drain. If you notice increased redness, swelling, warmth, pus or pain, call your surgeon.

4. Place two four-inch-by-four-inch sterile gauze pads on top of each other. Cut a two-inch slit in each dressing with clean scissors.

5. Place the dressing on the skin, where the tube comes out of your body, then place the drain tube within the slit.

6. Tape the dressings in place. Use paper first aid tape if you are allergic to adhesive tape.

7. Wash your hands again.

8. Safety-pin your drain to your blouse or underclothes. Always keep your drain below the level of your armpit.

Noting Sensory Changes

You are encouraged to touch your incision and scar, your chest and your underarm to experience the different sensations — or lack of sensations — you may find. You won't hurt yourself by doing this. This way, you'll find out which areas have lost feeling or are extremely sensitive to touch. You'll also find out what feels good to the touch and what doesn't.

As your incision heals, a scar will form. At first, the scar will be pink. Over time, the scar should fade. When you run your finger over the scar, you may notice that it has a firm ridge. This is called a healing ridge and it is normal. In time the ridge will soften. While the scar is healing, it may itch. Massaging vitamin E into the scar may make it feel more comfortable.

In the next year and a half, you will probably experience many different sensations in your chest, arm and underarm areas. If you know what to expect, these sensations won't be cause for worry.

Over the course of the first year or so, you may feel sharp pain, heaviness, stiffness, burning or a dull aching in your chest, arm, shoulder blade or rib cage on the side of your surgery. These sensations may vary. They may increase with tiredness, emotional stress or changes in the weather. These sensations will lessen in about a year.

Your incision, the scar as it forms, and the area around your scar will probably be permanently numb. This is because the breast's nerve supply has been cut. Occasionally, some sensation remains. It may feel like the tingling you get when your foot has been asleep and begins to wake up. This sensation may lessen over time.

If lymph nodes have been removed from under your armpit, some of the nerves there may be cut or stretched. As a result, you may feel an area of numbness or decreased feeling in your armpit and on the back of your arm. You may regain some or most of the sensation there.

Another sensation some women feel is that they still have their breast. This "phantom breast" experience is common. Some women find it disturbing, while others are comforted by it. Over time, the sensation lessens.

Exercising is Encouraged

Exercise is encouraged because it reduces stress and helps both your physical and emotional recovery. A gentle walking program is beneficial and appropriate, even for a woman who has not exercised for a number of years. When you walk, remember to stand up straight with your shoulders back.

If you have been involved in a strenuous exercise program before surgery, such as running, tennis, aerobics or weight-lifting, you will be able to get back to it in about six weeks. When you start up again, begin slowly. Before starting or resuming an exercise program, talk with your surgeon. For a specific exercise plan, ask your surgeon for a referral to a physical therapist.

Doing Specific Arm Exercises

*A*fter surgery, you may notice that when you move your arm, your chest, underarm area and shoulder may feel tight and sore. In time, you will recover full used of your arm, but you will have to work at regaining arm strength and flexibility. In six to eight weeks you should be able to:

- ◆ move your arm over your head

- ◆ move your arm out to your side

- ◆ touch the back of your neck

- ◆ touch the middle of your back

The following six-week exercise program has been designed to get you back to normal.

- ◆ The Arm Pumps and the stretching exercises should be done three times a day, every day. The weight lifting exercises should be done once a day, every other day.

- ◆ Try to reach farther each time you do the exercise. When you start to feel your incision pulling, stop and hold the stretch.

- ◆ Hold your stretches for at least 15 seconds. Do not bounce when stretching.

- ◆ In addition to stretching and weight lifting, you are encouraged to perform routine aerobic exercises, such as walking.

EXERCISE TO REDUCE SWELLING

Arm Pumps

Purpose: To increase lymphatic drainage. Start the day after surgery, and perform throughout your recovery if you notice swelling in your hand and/or your arm.

Position: Sit with your arm resting comfortably on pillows. Your arm should be higher than your heart.

Motion: While making a fist, bring your hand towards your shoulder. Take a deep breath; then straighten your arm, while relaxing your hand. Take a deep breath.

Repeat five times.

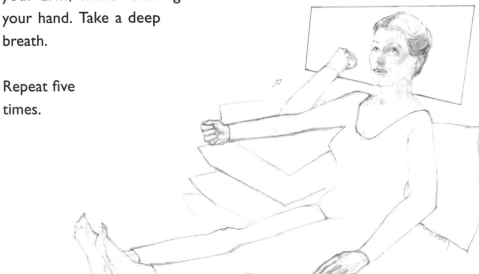

WEEKS ONE TO TWO (WHILE THE DRAIN IS IN)

Arm Raises I

Purpose: To keep your shoulder flexible.

Position: Stand, preferably in front of a mirror, with your arms by your side.

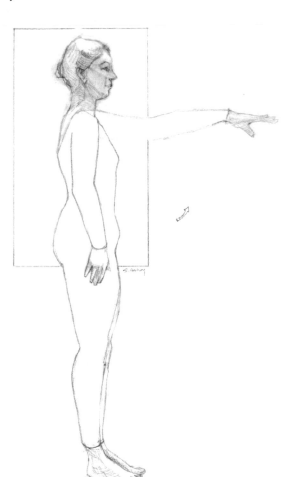

Motion: Keeping your arms straight; slowly raise both arms in front of you to shoulder level. Raise your arms only as far as you can without discomfort. Lower both arms.

Repeat five times.

Arm Raises 2

Purpose: To keep your shoulder flexible.

Position: Stand, preferably in front of a mirror, with your arms by your side.

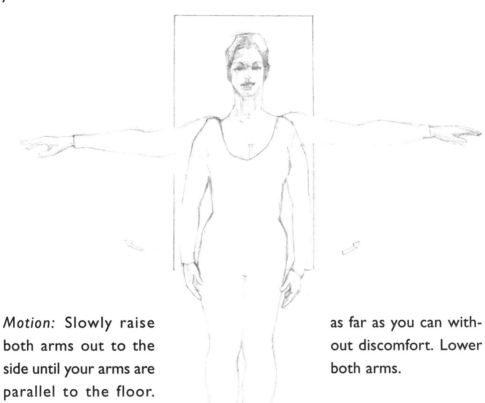

Motion: Slowly raise both arms out to the side until your arms are parallel to the floor. Raise your arms only as far as you can without discomfort. Lower both arms.

Repeat five times.

WEEKS TWO TO SIX (AFTER THE DRAIN IS REMOVED)

Back Climbing

Purpose: To help you reach the middle of your back with your affected arm.

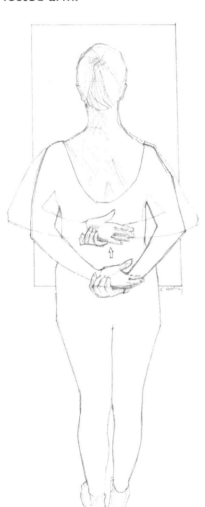

Position: Stand straight.

Motion: Place your hands behind your lower back and clasp them together. Slowly, slide your clasped hands up the center of your back. Stop when you start to feel your incision pulling. Hold that position for 15 seconds. Remember to breathe. Do once.

Clasp-Lift-Stretch

Purpose: To increase your overhead stretch.

Position: Stand or sit up straight with your feet on the floor.

Motion: 1. Clasp your hands together on your lap. Slowly raise your hands toward the ceiling. Make sure your arms are held straight. Stop when you feel your incision pulling. Hold that position for 15 seconds.

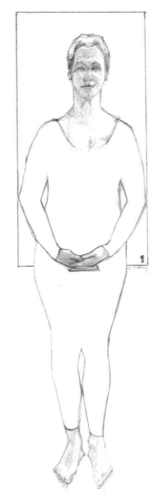

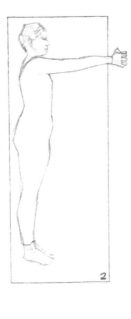

2. With your fingers still clasped, bend your arms and rest your hands on the top of your head. If the discomfort around your incision stops, con-

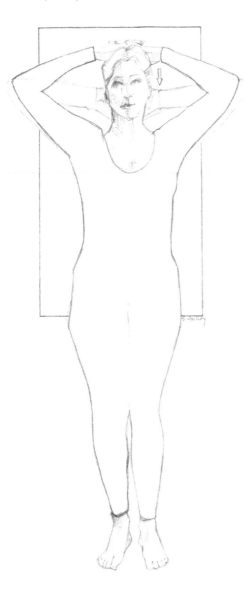

tinue sliding your clasped hands over your head until you reach the back of your neck. Keep your head upright.

3. Gradually stretch your elbows apart. Stretch only as far as you can without discomfort to your incision. Hold for 15 seconds.

4. Reverse the steps. Do once.

WEEKS FOUR TO SIX

Shoulder Stretch

Purpose: To stretch your underarm and the muscles in the back of your arm.

Position: Stand facing a wall, with your affected arm reaching up the wall as far as possible and your palm flat against the wall.

Motion: Lean forward until you feel a stretch in your underarm area. Hold for 15 seconds. As your ability to stretch improves, begin the exercise standing further away from the wall. Do once.

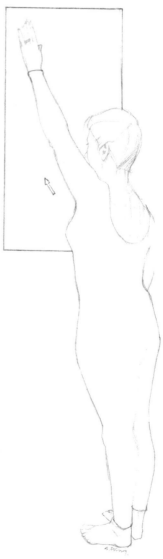

Corner Stretch

Purpose: To stretch your incision and chest muscles.

Position: Stand facing a corner. Brace the palms of your hands and forearms against the walls to each side of the corner.

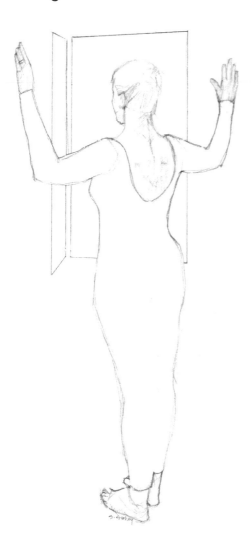

Motion: Slowly lean your chest in towards the corner. Keep your elbows at shoulder level and your forearms flat against the wall throughout the movement. You will feel the stretch across your chest wall. Hold this position for 15 seconds. Do once.

GENTLE WEIGHT LIFTING EXERCISES – WEEKS THREE TO SIX

*T*hese exercises require you to use weights to gently strengthen your arm muscles.

- ◆ Start off with one pound weights and slowly build up to three pounds. (You don't have to buy special equipment; you can use canned goods for your weights.)

- ◆ Do not exceed three pounds. If you have previously used heavier weights, ask your hospital physical therapist for some guidelines.

- ◆ Perform these exercises only once a day, every other day — your muscles need a day to repair themselves.

- ◆ Perform these exercises in front of a mirror so that you can check your form.

- ◆ It is important to breathe correctly when working with weights. You breathe out (exhale) when you work the muscle and you take a deep breath in (inhale) when you relax the muscle.

Shoulder Flexion

Purpose: To work the deltoid muscle, the muscle that raises the arm overhead.

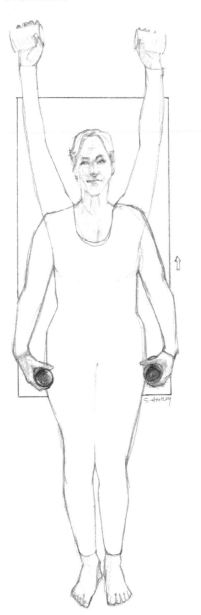

Position: Stand with your arms down by your sides, holding weights.

Motion: Keeping your arms straight, raise both of them over your head directly in front of your body. Exhale as you perform this motion. Go only as high as your involved shoulder will go. Lower both arms slowly. Inhale. Repeat 10 times.

Arm Bending

Purpose: To work the biceps muscle, the muscle which helps straighten the arm.

Position: Stand with your arms down by your sides, holding weights.

Motion: Bend your arms, bringing your hands towards your shoulder. Exhale as you perform this motion. Slowly return to your starting position. Inhale. Repeat 10 times.

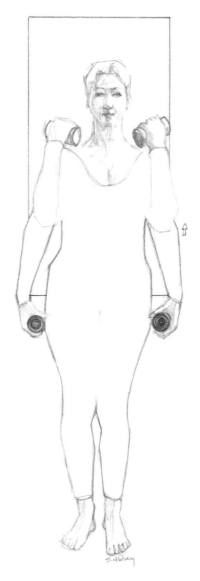

Arm Extension

Purpose: To work the triceps muscle, the muscle which helps straighten the arm.

Position: Lie on your back. With a weight in your hand, bend your arm so that your elbow points up towards the ceiling. Hold your arm still with your opposite hand.

Motion: Slowly straighten your arm until it is fully extended. Exhale as you perform this motion. Slowly return to your starting position. Inhale. Repeat 10 times with each arm.

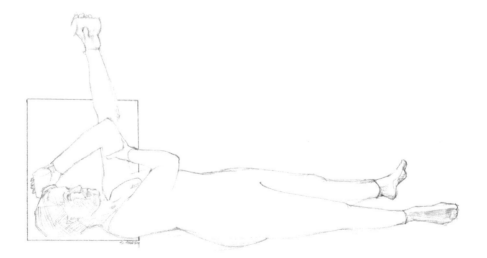

AFTER SIX WEEKS

After six weeks, you are usually able to resume all previous activities. In addition to stretching and weight lifting, you are encouraged to do regular aerobic exercise.

You may choose to do these exercises by yourself or get some professional instruction. Many women do better with individual instruction from a physical therapist. If you feel assistance would help, ask your surgeon for a referral to the physical therapy department connected with your hospital.

Preventing Lymphedema: Special Nail, Hand and Arm Care

After surgery, there is no reason why you can't use your hand and arm in a normal way, and enjoy doing all the things you did before the surgery. However, you will need to give some special attention to your nails, hand and arm on the side of your surgery, to prevent a possible complication called lymphedema. Lymphedema is a chronic swelling of the hand and/or arm.

In a modified radical mastectomy, the lymph nodes under the arm next to the affected breast are removed. The removal of these underarm lymph nodes (axillary lymph nodes) can cause the lymphatic draining system (primarily made up of lymph nodes, lymph vessels and lymph fluid) in your affected hand and arm to become sluggish. Since this system is an important part of your overall immune system and helps keep infections in check, this sluggishness increases the risk of infection in the affected side. An injury or an untreated infection of your affected hand, arm or underarm area may lead to chronic swelling or lymphedema.

Although lymphedema can and should be treated, it cannot be cured. Lymphedema may develop soon after surgery or many years later. If swelling does develop, it is important to start treatment as soon as possible.

The following guidelines will help you prevent lymphedema:

Stay physically active. If you haven't been physically active or haven't regularly done physical exercises, it is important to gradually build up your physical stamina. General physical activity, such as walking, is a good beginning. Physical activity causes the muscles throughout your body to contract, and this encourages lymphatic drainage. Building muscle strength in both arms also is desirable, since good muscle tone is a safeguard against injuring your arm. Many times, a woman will injure her arm by carrying a seemingly light package or briefcase that turns out to be too heavy for her.

Protect your nails, hand, arm and underarm from injury. Injury can lead to an infection as well as chronic swelling. Give yourself gentle manicures; don't cut your cuticles and avoid artificial nails — they are a source of fungal infections. Bring your own manicuring tools to your manicurist, if you have your nails done professionally. Wear protective gloves while performing jobs that might lead to injury, such as home maintenance, yard work, and baking. Wear long-sleeved clothes, insect repellent and sun screen to protect against sunburn and insect bites. Last, use an electric razor if you shave under your arms.

If you injure your hand or arm, treat the injury appropriately. Vigorously wash the wound with soap and warm water several times a day. Cover the wound and keep it dry. If the injury looks like it's getting infected (i.e., red, swelling, pus or pain), see your doctor immediately for antibiotic therapy.

Tips to Avoid Injuring Your Hand and Arm

◆ Avoid carrying heavy objects on the affected side, such as hand-bags, briefcases, or suitcases.

◆ Avoid having blood drawn, injections or chemotherapy in the affected arm.

◆ Avoid acupuncture in the affected arm.

◆ Avoid having blood pressure taken in the affected arm.

5.

Getting Back To Your Normal Routines

Bathing and Showering

You may take a bath as soon as you want. However, if you have a dressing over your incision, do not get it wet. To make sure you don't get your dressing wet, you may need help while bathing; or you might choose to take a sponge bath. If you have a drain, don't submerge your chest under water.

After your drain has been removed by your surgeon, you're free to shower. At first, stand with your back to the shower head to avoid the full force of the water on your incision. It's okay if your steri-strips get wet; just pat them dry with a towel. Don't be afraid to touch your incision. You will not hurt anything. Since it will be numb, it may feel funny — as if you're washing someone else.

Sleeping

Most people find it difficult to sleep during their hospital stay. Once at home, you will probably return to your normal sleep pattern. It is alright to sleep in any position you find comfortable. Many women find that lying on their back, with pillows under their affected arm, is the most comfortable position. If you have any problem sleeping, try the following:

◆ Cut out beverages with caffeine (coffee, tea, soda, chocolate) five hours before bedtime.

◆ Take your prescribed pain medication twenty minutes before bedtime.

◆ Drink some chamomile tea or warm milk at bedtime.

◆ Take a warm bath. Remember not to get your dressing wet, submerge your drain, nor soak your incision until a week after surgery.

Eating Healthy

Your diet is an important part of your recovery. Eating the right kinds of food during your treatment can help you feel better and stay stronger. A nutritious diet always is essential for your body to work most effectively. For people with cancer, good nutrition is especially vital:

◆ A healthy diet can help you keep up your strength, prevent body tissue from breaking down, and rebuild tissues that cancer treatment may harm.

◆ People who eat well during their treatment are better able to cope with the side effects of treatment.

When you are unable to eat enough food or the right kinds of food, your body uses stored nutrients as a source of energy. As a result, your natural defenses (your immune system) are weakened and your body isn't as effective in fighting infection. This defense system is especially important to you at this time.

Try to eat a variety of foods every day. No one food or group of foods contains all the nutrients you need. A diet designed to keep your body strong will include daily servings from these food groups:

◆ Fruits and Vegetables: Raw or cooked vegetables, fruits, and fruit juices provide vitamins and minerals the body needs.

◆ Protein: Protein helps your body heal itself and fight infection. Fish, poultry, eggs, cheese, beans and lean meat are rich in protein.

◆ Grains: Bread, pasta, and cereals provide carbohydrates and B vitamins. Carbohydrates provide a good source of energy.

◆ Dairy: Low-fat milk and other dairy products provide protein, vitamins and calcium.

Try to drink eight 8-ounce glasses of liquid a day. The following liquids can be included if tolerated: water, fruit juice, herbal tea, non-caffeinated tonic, and milk.

Beverages that contain caffeine or alcohol are not included in the above list because they are mildly dehydrating. A moderate amount of caffeinated beverages and/or alcohol can be drunk, if you can tolerate them.

Managing Weight Gain

You may find that you gain weight during treatment, though you are eating the same amount as before your surgery. It's important not to go on a low calorie or crash diet if you notice a weight gain. Instead, tell your doctor so you can find out what may be causing this change.

Some anti-cancer drugs, such as prednisone, lead to weight gain by causing the body to retain fluid. The extra weight is in the form of water and doesn't mean you are eating too much. Your surgeon or medical oncologist may recommend limiting the salt you eat and increasing your intake of water, since salt causes your body to hold on to water and water dilutes the salt. Your surgeon or medical oncologist may instruct you to continue eating a balanced diet, but to choose foods that are low in fat.

You also may be encouraged to increase your exercise level. Activities such as walking and swimming are good options, even if you have not exercised regularly in a while. If you feel you need some help with your diet and nutritional concerns, ask your surgeon to refer you to a registered dietician.

Taking Care of Constipation

During the first few days at home, some women find that they are troubled by constipation. Temporary constipation can be the result of anesthesia, pain medication and/or inactivity. The following are a few suggestions that should get you back to normal and keep you regular:

◆ Drink 10 glasses of liquid a day. The following liquids can be included if tolerated: water, fruit juice, herbal tea, non-caffeinated tonic, and milk. Caffeinated coffee, tea, sodas and alcohol shouldn't be counted as liquids because they are mildly dehydrating. However, some women find that a cup of coffee or tea in the morning helps bring on a bowel movement.

◆ Increase the fiber in your diet with bran cereals, fruits and vegetables.

◆ Practice some form of physical activity each day.

◆ Eat prunes or drink prune juice. This also helps you move your bowels.

*N*ote: The section on nutrition was adapted from a book entitled, *Eating Hints and Recipes and Tips for Better Nutrition During Cancer Treatment.* It can be obtained, free of charge, from the National Institute of Health.

Driving

You can begin driving again when you feel ready and when you are no longer taking narcotic pain medication. Turning the wheel and/or parallel parking may feel uncomfortable, but you won't injure your surgery site when you do so. The type of car you drive (power steering versus manual steering) also will affect how comfortable it is to drive.

Going Back To Work

Going back to work is based on a number of factors and should be decided after a discussion with your surgeon. Some important considerations will be: how physically and emotionally demanding and stressful your job is; how much you want to return to work; how fast you are healing; and whether or not you are going to need further therapy (i.e., radiation and chemotherapy).

Should you tell your co-workers that you have had a mastectomy? This question is important, not because you should be embarrassed about having breast cancer, but for practical reasons. Under the Federal Rehabilitation Act of 1973, federal employers or companies receiving federal funding cannot discriminate against cancer survivors. But state laws vary and federal legislation doesn't affect the private sector.

If your co-workers know your medical history, you may risk overt discrimination, as well as more subtle discrimination. So, some women choose to keep quiet about their mastectomy at work. There is a catch, however. If no one knows about your surgery, you can't get the support you may need. This is a difficult situation that does not have an easy answer. You need to do what feels right for you.

6.

Considering Breast Forms (Breast Prosthesis)

Generally, you will be able to wear the same clothes as you did before surgery. After your drains come out, try to wear clothes that button or zip up the back. When you reach up and back to button or zip, the stretch will help you regain flexibility in your shoulder and arm.

If you wear loose clothes, you may feel comfortable and attractive without padding. If you wear form-fitting clothes, you may consider wearing padding. Some women choose to go without padding, in loose or form-fitting clothes, and that's a perfectly valid choice. Some women drape a scarf over their chest as an attractive accessory and a way to conceal the surgery without using padding.

Temporary Breast Forms

If you wish, a lightweight temporary breast form can be worn immediately after surgery. Your first breast form should be made of a soft, lightweight material. It can be safety-pinned to your underclothes (i.e., camisole, undershirt, slip). When it's comfortable to wear a bra, you can place the breast form in your bra cup. You will need to safety-pin it in place.

You have several options for your first temporary breast form: you can make one yourself; you can get a complimentary form from the American Cancer Society; or you can buy one.

MAKING YOUR OWN TEMPORARY BREAST FORM

You can make a temporary form by using a foam rubber or a cloth-covered shoulder pad; or when it's comfortable to wear a bra, you can put soft lamb's wool in your bra cup. The lamb's wool can be purchased at your pharmacy.

BUYING A TEMPORARY BREAST FORM

The Softee is a specially-designed camisole with built-in detachable breast forms. As its name suggests, it is a soft and comfortable undergarment. Individual inner pockets securely hold the breast form in place, on one or both sides. You can wear the Softee home from the hospzital and continue wearing it until you get a more permanent form. To find out where to purchase a Softee, see "Resources" section under "Appearance".

Manufacturers of permanent breast forms also make temporary ones. They cost about eight dollars. They can be washed by hand and allowed to dry. See the next section on permanent breast forms to find out where you can buy one.

GETTING A COMPLIMENTARY TEMPORARY BREAST FORM

The American Cancer Society (ACS) will be happy to give you a temporary breast form through a program called "Reach For Recovery." The program's specially-trained volunteers are women who have had breast cancer surgery. They will visit you in the hospital or at home and bring the breast form. Call your local ACS chapter for more information.

Permanent Breast Forms

In about three to six weeks after surgery, when your incision is well-healed and comfortable to touch, you can be fitted for a more permanent and durable breast form. This permanent breast form lasts from one to five years, feels natural, looks good in form-fitting clothes, and replaces the weight of your breast.

The most natural of these forms is made of a silicone gel, with a polyurethane surface. So, when you get and give hugs, the silicone form gives and feels like your own breast.

A permanent breast form is deliberately weighted to prevent your bra from riding up on your chest. It also provides a balanced weight between the right and left sides of your chest. This is important, since an imbalance can lead to problems with posture, as well as neck, back and shoulder pain. The breast form may feel heavy at first. In time, it will come to feel more natural.

Permanent breast forms come in a variety of shapes, weights, skin tones and sizes. Working with a good fitter, you should find one that is right for you.

NO-BRA BREAST FORMS

Generally, breast forms are held in place by a bra. But there is a new breast form that is securely held against your chest with a non-irritating adhesive. You place a special adhesive-backed strip on your chest (it can remain on for a week). Then, just press on the breast form. It works much like a velcro fastener. You may remove the form at any time or keep it on 24 hours a day. You also can wear it in the shower, sauna or when you swim.

Caring for Your Permanent Breast Form

*W*ith proper care, your permanent breast form should last a number of years. The following tips will help make sure it does last:

◆ Hand-wash the form each day in warm, soapy water, using a mild soap. Rinse the form in warm water and blot it dry with a soft towel. Never use harsh cleaners or chemicals on your breast form. Never dry it over heat.

◆ Keep your breast form stored in its original box (in its "cradle") when not in use.

◆ Avoid puncture holes from pins, sharp jewelry or cat claws.

Will My Insurance Pay for a Breast Form?

*I*f you choose to wear a breast form, your medical insurance should pay for one breast form for each breast, and two bras, every one to two years. When you purchase your form, you will be asked to pay for it out-of-pocket. You will need to submit a form to your insurance company to be reimbursed. It is important to ask your surgeon (or any of your doctors) for a prescription for a "breast prosthesis", and another for "two surgical bras." Make sure you submit your prescription and your receipts to your insurance company. Forms range in price from about $175.00 to $450.00.

BRAS AND FITTING

The first week after surgery, you may find it more comfortable to wear an undershirt or camisole next to your skin, rather than a bra. If and when you feel ready to wear your regular bra, you may notice that your chest is temporarily swollen, and you may not be able to fasten your bra. If so, you may need to buy a bra expander, which extends the hook-and-eye section of your bra. You can buy one in the lingerie section of most department stores.

The key to a well-fitted breast form is a well-fitted bra. Most women wear the wrong bra size — either too large or too tight. Allow a professional fitter to measure you and help you find a bra that is the correct size and fit.

Most permanent breast forms can be worn with any well-fitted bra. You may be able to wear the same bra you've always worn, even your underwire bra. However, some women prefer special bras that have pockets to hold the breast form in place. These bras can be quite pretty and come in a variety of colors. Some of the features of a bra that provides good support and comfort are:

◆ wide shoulder straps

◆ wide band below the cup

◆ wide band around your back

◆ multiple hooks-and-eyes to fasten it

As mentioned, your medical insurance will reimburse you for the purchase of your bra. Just ask the salesperson to write "surgical bra" on the sales receipt. Remember that any of your doctors can give you a prescription for a "surgical bra." Any well-fitted bra can be considered a "surgical bra."

Tips for Fitting

- ◆ Call ahead to make an appointment so that you can be sure you'll be taken care of by an experienced fitter.

- ◆ When you arrive for your appointment, ask for your fitter by name, so that you can be taken care of discreetly.

- ◆ Allow adequate time for your fitting. A trained fitter may need up to one hour to properly fit you.

- ◆ Wear or bring along a well-fitted, favorite garment. This way, you and the fitter can see your contours clearly.

- ◆ Once fitted, your breast forms should feel comfortable, look natural in your bra and clothes, and remain in place when you move.

How to Find an Experienced Fitter

◆ The "Reach For Recovery" coordinator of your local chapter of the American Cancer Society has a resource list of experienced fitters.

◆ Better department stores usually carry breast forms in the lingerie department and have experienced fitters to help you.

◆ Surgical or medical supply stores often carry breast forms. However, this is a very clinical setting, which may not be to your liking. Before deciding whether or not to go, call the surgical supply store and speak to their fitter. If you find the fitter to be a knowledgeable and caring person, the clinical setting shouldn't matter as much. To find such stores, look in the Yellow Pages under "Surgical Appliances and Supplies."

Breast Reconstruction

Most women are good candidates for breast reconstruction. As already noted on page 6, breast reconstruction is a surgical procedure performed by a plastic surgeon during which the breast contour is rebuilt, and if the woman desires, the areola and nipple as well. Breast reconstruction may be done at the time of the mastectomy (immediate reconstruction) or at any time afterwards. If you are interested in reconstruction, ask your surgeon for a referral to a plastic surgeon.

7.

Your Emotional Recovery

Taking Care of Your Feelings

You will need to make your own needs and feelings your top priority during the course of your diagnosis, treatment and recovery. Though this may sound obvious, it may be difficult to do. Many women are used to putting other people's needs — those of children, partners, friends — ahead of their own. Women who easily help others find it difficult to ask for help for themselves. Yet, taking care of yourself and reaching out to people who can provide you with support is essential to getting well. Your emotional recovery should be as deliberate as your physical recovery.

Be kind to yourself. Treat yourself to activities that make you feel good and give you pleasure. They don't necessarily have to cost a lot of money. Walking in the park, sitting on your porch, taking care of your plants or garden, sitting in a warm bath, or getting a massage can be very comforting. Try to let go of activities and responsibilities that are physically and emotionally draining. Set priorities. Do those things that give you satisfaction; try to let go of the "oughts" and "shoulds."

Be honest with yourself. In order to receive support from others, you need to know what you want and need from them. This is a time to look inward; it's a time to explore your feelings, needs and desires. Then, you must have the strength to communicate those needs and feelings in as direct and honest a manner as possible.

Selecting Your Support Team

SEEK OUT FAMILY AND FRIENDS

*F*amily and friends can be a wonderful source of support and help. However, sometimes they don't know what to say or do. Help them comfort you.

- ◆ Let them know they don't have to say anything; all they need to do is just be there — to sit with you, to listen to you, to let you cry.

- ◆ Ask them to help with meals, to run errands, to care for your children, to drive you or come with you to appointments. Some people feel more comfortable showing their support by "doing" rather than talking or listening.

Not everyone is able to give you the support and understanding you need in the way that you need it. Some of your friends, co-workers and family, no matter how well-meaning, can make you feel worse rather than better. Sometimes, a close friend or relative will become cold or distant when you tell them about your breast cancer. In extreme cases, they may literally disappear from your life. Often, they have an irrational fear of cancer. Although their absence may be very painful to you and may feel like a personal rejection, remember, they are reacting to their fear of cancer, not to their feelings about you.

Join a Support Group

A strong remedy for dealing with painful experiences is to be able to talk to others who are going through similar experiences. During treatment and recovery, it's particularly helpful to talk with other women who have breast cancer. Most of them, like yourself, have experienced a range of strong and often scary emotions such as fear, depression and anger. Seeing others express emotions similar to yours will help you realize that your own feelings are normal.

A support group provides understanding, strength and companionship; it becomes a safe place to express feelings that you can't or won't share with family or friends. Whether you have family or not, the group becomes a "family" of special friends.

Each support group has its own personality — made unique by the women who participate in it. If you go to a support group meeting and it isn't a good fit, don't be discouraged. Try another support group; it's worth it. Many women feel that their support group was vital to their emotional recovery.

To find a support group, ask your surgeon or hospital social worker, or call some of the organizations listed in the Resource section.

FIND ONE-TO-ONE SUPPORT

You may feel most comfortable talking with another breast cancer survivor in a one-to-one situation. One source to which you can turn is the American Cancer Society's "Reach for Recovery" program. The program provides emotional support and information through trained volunteers who have had breast cancer surgery. If you wish, a volunteer can call or visit you at the hospital or at your home. To get in touch with a volunteer, call your local chapter of the American Cancer Society.

Another way to get in touch with a breast cancer survivor is to talk with your doctors, your hospital social worker or your clergy about putting you in contact with someone. If there are women's organizations or breast cancer advocacy groups in your city or town, you might want to check with them for referrals.

CONSIDER PROFESSIONAL EMOTIONAL SUPPORT

Sometimes, talking with your family, friends or your support group may not be enough. At such times, talking with a caring mental health professional can be very helpful, since they are specifically trained to focus on your needs. Having private and confidential conversations with a trained professional can help you sort out issues around self-esteem, your feelings about the changes in your body, your anxiety and fears, really any personal issues that concern you. They can also provide expert guidance on ways to cope with issues and problems that come up with your partner, children, friends and family.

You can consult with a variety of resource people: for personal concerns, a clinical psychologist, nurse therapist, clinical social worker, or psychiatrist; for marital and family issues, a marriage and family counselor; for sexual concerns, a certified sexual counselor. Ask your doctors and hospital social worker for referrals.

TALK WITH YOUR CHILDREN

You may be tempted to protect your children, and maybe yourself, by not telling them about your operation. However, children — even very young children — can sense when something is wrong. Usually it's better to be honest and involve your children in your recovery process from the beginning. Tell them the truth — simply and in a manner and language appropriate to their age level.

How do you know what is age appropriate? You'll find out by encouraging questions from them. Your children will ask you what they need to know, when they are ready to know it. Give them the information they ask for, not more. Children absorb stressful information in stages. After they have time to internalize the information you've given them, they will ask more questions when they are ready. Give your children permission to ask any question, and explain that it's more scary when they don't ask — because their imagination fills in the gaps.

If you want some help talking with your children, ask your surgeon, family doctor, or hospital social worker to set up a consultation with a health care professional who works specifically with children, who can speak to you alone or meet with you and your family.

Physical and Sexual Intimacy

Resuming, maintaining or starting a satisfying sexual relationship is an important part of your emotional recovery. A mastectomy can cause a woman to doubt her attractiveness, and a loving touch can go a long way towards helping a woman regain sexual self-confidence.

You may not be ready for sexual intimacy; but you may want and need to be touched and hugged without the pressure to go further. Sometimes, even without noticing it, couples drift apart physically; they stop their loving routines, such as cuddling in front of the television or hugging each other.

Notice if this is happening between you and your partner. If it is, make sure to get touch back into your relationship. Holding hands, asking for or giving a hug, stroking an arm or back all "remind" you and your partner how important touch is.

Sometimes, a neck and back massage also is very comforting and an intimate experience that can bring pleasure to both of you, without any pressure to go further. To make it more comfortable, you can either lie on your unaffected side or sit up. Use lotion or oil, and warm it by rubbing it between the palms of the hands.

You may find that both you and your partner have less interest in sex than you did before your diagnosis. This is quite common and normal. The stress of diagnosis and treatment, along with the many strong emotions you're probably feeling, can reduce sexual desire. It's difficult to feel romantic when you and your partner are trying to cope with anger, fear, depression, anxiety and other strong feelings. Talking about these feelings can encourage intimacy; and intimacy can create romance and sexual interest.

In time, you should find your sexual desire returning to the level it was before diagnosis. If your interest doesn't seem to be returning, ask the doctor with whom you feel most comfortable for a referral to a counselor specially trained to talk with you about sexual intimacy. A certified sex therapist can help you figure out the causes of low sexual desire and suggest steps that can lead to improved sexual satisfaction.

RESUMING YOUR SEXUAL RELATIONS

*R*esuming your sexual relations may be intimidating. There may be some awkward moments. There is also the potential for misunderstanding and hurt feelings. As with all other aspects of your emotional recovery, it's important for you to be honest with yourself about your needs, concerns and fears, and to be able to talk with your partner about them. It may help if you can start these conversations.

Sometimes, partners assume that you shouldn't have sex for some time after surgery. Partners commonly fear that love-making will hurt you, so they may seem hesitant. Women often misinterpret this as rejection. You can prevent this potential misunderstanding by talking frankly with your partner. You can reassure your partner that love-making won't harm your incision and that it isn't bad for your health; and they can reassure you that they still love and desire you.

Whenever you and your partner feel ready to have sexual relations, you may find the following helpful:

◆ Wear something that makes you feel comfortable and desirable, like a pretty camisole, nightie or negligee.

◆ Your incision and chest may be tender, numb or particularly sensitive to touch. Many women don't enjoy having the area over the incision caressed; others do. It's important to let your partner know this — and whatever else — does and doesn't feel good.

◆ There is no right or wrong position for having sex. Whatever position is comfortable for you is the "right" one. Women report that one of the most comfortable positions is with their partner on top. This position puts the least amount of pressure on your chest, especially if partners use their arms for support above you.

◆ Try laying with your affected arm over your incision, so that your hand is resting on your unaffected shoulder. You can also place a small pillow over or under your arm, to further protect your incision. This may help you feel your incision is safe and will allow you to relax.

◆ Tamoxifen, chemotherapy and/or menopause may cause vaginal dryness. This can interfere with sexual enjoyment. There are a number of good, non-prescription products you can buy to provide vaginal lubrication, for example, Replense, Probe, and Astroglide. Replense is good because it's routinely applied and needn't be timed with intercourse. It should be applied once in the morning, three times a week. Probe and Astroglide are used as lubricants during intercourse.

You may find that talking to your partner about sex is not easy to do. You're not alone. Many find it difficult to talk openly about sexual matters. If you're having difficulty, a specially trained and certified sex therapist can be of great help. Ask any of your doctors, your hospital social worker or your personal counselor for a referral.

Tips for Talking About Sexual Intimacy

◆ Set aside a time to talk to each other about sexual intimacy.

◆ Find a time when there are no distractions, the television is off, and the children are asleep — time for just the two of you.

◆ Talk to each other in a sexually "neutral" area, not in a place where you are sexually intimate.

◆ Try to talk to each other honestly and with humor.

SINGLE WOMEN AND SEXUAL INTIMACY

If you are a single woman, you may have some special concerns about physical intimacy. One concern you may have is when and how to tell friends and lovers that you have been diagnosed with cancer and have had breast surgery. It can be helpful to talk to other single women who have had breast cancer to find out how they coped, as well as to receive and give emotional support. Ask your friends, hospital social worker, doctors, clergy and the "Reach for Recovery" coordinator to put you in touch with other single women. There are two wonderful books that address the particular concerns of single women: *Up Front: Sex and the Post-Mastectomy Woman* by Linda Dackman, and *Invisible Scars* by Mimi Greenberg, Ph.D.

Whether single or with a partner, it's important to know what you do and don't want and need for yourself. This knowledge will ease recovery for you and for those who love you.

8.

Your Treatment Plan

No Further Treatment

After the mastectomy, some women will need no further treatment. Careful follow-up is important and means regular clinical examinations and mammograms (special x-rays of your breast). Some of the questions you will need to ask your surgeon are:

- ◆ How often do I need to return for examinations?

- ◆ How often do I need to have a mammogram?

- ◆ What other kinds of tests do I need to have, and how often do they need to be done?

Other Treatments

Your surgeon may suggest the use of other forms of treatment, such as tamoxifen, chemotherapy and radiation therapy in addition to your mastectomy. To find out what is the best personal treatment, you may want to talk to several specialists such as a medical oncologist, a doctor who treats cancer with medication and a radiation oncologist, a doctor who treats cancer with radiation therapy. You may also find that a second opinion is useful in providing additional information.

The decision to have further treatment can be a difficult one for you and your doctors to make. Various factors need to be taken into account, including a careful analysis of the tissue removed in surgery. Other tests, like a bone scan, chest x-rays and blood work, to name a few, may also be needed. As important are your feelings about undergoing further treatment. These feelings and concerns should be carefully discussed with your doctors.

Some of the factors considered in making a treatment decision are:

◆ *Tumor size:* The size of the cancer in the breast.

◆ *Lymph node status:* The presence or absence of cancer cells in the lymph nodes under the arm on the side of the mastectomy.

◆ *Histology:* What the cancer looks like under the microscope, the type of breast cancer it is, and whether it is slow or fast-growing.

◆ *Hormone assay tests:* Whether the tumor responds to the hormones, estrogen and progesterone.

◆ *DNA Analysis:* Computer analysis of the chromosome content of the tumor to determine if the cancer is slow or fast-growing.

◆ *Your thoughts and feelings:* How you feel about further treatment and the nature and effects of that treatment.

At first, these tests and their results may seem a bit technical. But don't be put off. If you're interested, your surgeon, medical oncologist, or oncology nurse will be happy to carefully explain what these tests mean in terms of your treatment. In addition, there are a number of good books and pamphlets that explain the nature of these tests in a clear and understandable manner. *Dr. Susan Love's Breast Book* by Susan M. Love, M.D. is particularly helpful.

Hormonal Therapy

Tamoxifen (Novadex) is the most common oral medication that is given to reduce the risk of the cancer coming back. Some breast cancer cells "like" estrogen. A woman's body makes estrogen both before and after menopause. Of course, after menopause your body produces less estrogen. When a woman takes tamoxifen, the drug "attaches" itself to cancer cells that may be in the body and prevents them from growing.

Tamoxifen is generally well-tolerated. However, some women do report experiencing hot flashes, vaginal dryness, vaginal discharge, weight gain and depression. While taking tamoxifen, you should get a regular pap smear and pelvic examination, as there is a slight increase in the risk of uterine cancer. Tamoxifen can be prescribed and monitored by your surgeon or medical oncologist. Some questions you may want to ask these doctors are:

◆ What are the risks and benefits of taking tamoxifen?

◆ How long do I need to take it?

◆ How often do I need to have a pap smear and pelvic examination?

◆ Do I need any other tests on a regular basis if I take tamoxifen?

◆ What are some other possible side effects of tamoxifen?

Chemotherapy

Chemotherapy is planned and supervised by a medical oncologist. It is medication that kills cancer cells. It is usually a combination of medications that can be given orally and/or intravenously. Chemotherapy can be given on an out-patient basis or during a hospital stay. The possible side effects include fatigue, nausea, low white blood cell count, hair loss and the onset of menopause. Medical oncologists and oncology nurses are sensitive to the fears you may have about chemotherapy and will work with you to help reduce the side effects. Once you are referred to a medical oncologist, there are a number of questions you may want to ask:

◆ What medications do you suggest?

◆ How effective are these drugs in cases similar to mine?

◆ What are the risks and benefits?

◆ How long will I be on chemotherapy?

◆ What can be done to reduce the side effects?

◆ Will I be able to work while on chemotherapy?

◆ How often will I need to see you after treatment ends?

Radiation Therapy

Radiation therapy is planned and supervised by a radiation oncologist. Radiation therapy is a series of daily treatments that take less than 5 minutes and are painless. The most common temporary side effects are a sun burn-like redness to the skin and fatigue. When you meet with the radiation oncologist you may want to ask some of the following questions:

◆ How long will the daily treatments last and how long will I be in the radiation therapy department each day?

◆ How many weeks will the treatments take?

◆ What are the risks and benefits?

◆ What are the common side effects?

◆ What can be done to reduce the side effects?

◆ How often will I need to see you after treatment ends?

Regular Follow-Up

After your treatment ends, you will have frequent clinical examinations and routine mammograms. During the first two years, you will see your doctors every three to six months. Since you may have several doctors; for example, a surgeon, a medical oncologist, and your primary doctor, you will need to check with each to see whom you will visit, and when.

The time after treatment ends and between doctors' visits can be an anxious one. Having gone through a diagnosis of breast cancer, a mastectomy and post-surgery treatment, it's no wonder that any physical discomfort you have, such as a headache or a cough, might cause you to be anxious, and to have thoughts of a recurrence. The best way to assure yourself that you are okay is to discuss your observations and concerns with your doctors.

Breast Self-Examination

You are encouraged to perform a monthly breast self-examination (BSE), in addition to having clinical breast examinations by your health care provider and mammograms.

You may find that when you examine yourself, you become anxious about finding a new lump, or even sad because it brings up your recent experience with breast cancer. You may also feel uncertain about what you are looking or feeling for. These reactions are common and understandable. Talking with your doctor, your social worker, or other breast cancer survivors about these feelings can help you deal with them. Asking for individual instruction in BSE can help you feel more confident about your skills.

Also, it can be helpful to think about BSE in a new light. Think of BSE as a way to get familiar with your new body, not a way to "find cancer." Make BSE a positive affirmation of your health. After you examine yourself, you could say to yourself, "My chest and breast look healthy; my chest and breast feel healthy; my chest and breast are healthy."

How to do BSE

If you continue to menstruate, the best time to do BSE is seven to ten days after the first day of your cycle. This is the time during your menstrual cycle when the breast is least tender to touch. Remember, if you had pre-menstrual breast tenderness before your mastectomy, you will probably continue to feel that discomfort in your remaining breast. Discomfort that comes and goes with your period is not a sign of breast cancer. If you no longer menstruate, pick a day, such as the first day of the month, to do BSE.

A breast examination has two parts, the visual exam and the palpation (touch) exam. During the visual examination, you will look at yourself in a mirror. During the palpation exam, you will use your hand to examine yourself. If you find any changes, show them to your doctors.

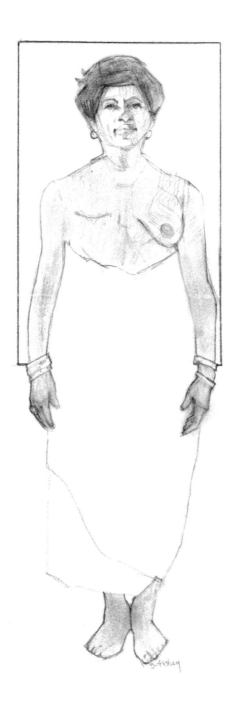

The Visual Examination

*S*tand in front of a mirror. Hold your hands (palm side down) in front of you. Compare your unaffected hand to your affected hand. Notice if you have any swelling in your affected hand.

Then with your arms at your side, look in the mirror and compare the size of your arms. Do you notice any swelling? If so, you may be developing lymphedema and should make an appointment to begin treatment.

Next, with arms at your side, stand and examine your whole chest area from your collarbone to your bra line, and from the middle of your chest to your underarm area.

Raise your hands above your head. Slowly, turn from side to side, so that you can examine from the middle of your chest to your underarm area. If you notice any of the following changes, show them to your doctor:

◆ Persistent rash, redness, or discoloration on your scar, chest and/or breast.

◆ Persistent itchy rash on your nipple or areola.

◆ Nipple discharge that is spontaneous and persistent.

◆ A change in the size or shape of your breast, such as a dimple.

◆ A lump in your breast, chest and/or scar.

The Palpation Examination

*D*uring the palpation examination, you will use your hands to examine yourself.

Lie on your back and use your opposite hand to examine yourself. For example, if you are examining your right side, use your left hand.

If your breast size is a B cup or larger, the following position will spread your breast tissue evenly over your chest. Turn on your side with your knees bent, as if you were going to sleep on your side; then turn your upper body away from your bent knees, so that your chest faces the ceiling.

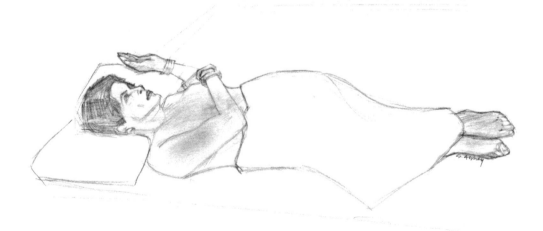

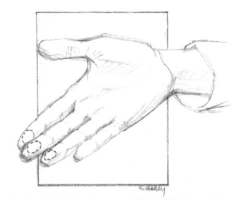

Hold your hand flat and use the fleshy pads of your middle three fingers, rather than the tips.

At each spot you examine, move the pads of your fingers in three small circles — about the size of a dime. Use three levels of pressure — light, medium and deep. When pressing deeply, try to feel your ribs. Your ribs feel like a washboard.

A good examination pattern is the "vertical strip method." Always start in your armpit and examine down towards your bra line.

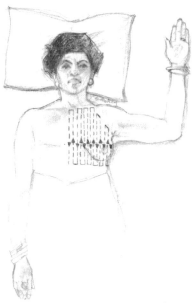

When you examine the side of your mastectomy, pay particular attention to your scar. If you notice a hard lump, a thickening or any change, show it to your doctor.

Individual Instruction in BSE

Most women benefit from individual instruction in BSE. Individual instruction will teach you how to hold your hand, how deeply to press, how to know what your ribs feel like, and how to sort out a lump from the normal lumpy feeling of your breast.

Ask your doctor or nurse to spend some time with you reviewing BSE. You may also check with your doctors or hospital to see if there is a nurse who can teach you BSE.

The Mammatech Corporation has developed an effective step-by-step home teaching program that includes a life-like breast model and a 45-minute videotape. The breast model helps you distinguish a lump from the normal lumpy feeling of the breast.

Remember, you are the best judge of your own body — don't ever be embarrassed to bring a change or concern to the attention of your nurse or doctor.

9.

In Conclusion

*E*ach day, it may be helpful for you to remind yourself that you are not alone. Over 100,000 women in this country have a mastectomy every year. These women have found in themselves and through others the strength and resources to recover and heal. Think of this community of survivors; tell yourself that you are not alone; affirm each day your belief that you, too, will recover and heal. We hope that this guide has contributed to your recovery and healing.

Appendices

Glossary

areola: The darker part of the breast surrounding the nipple.

axilla: The armpit area that contains lymph nodes, lymph and blood vessels, fat and muscles.

axillary lymph nodes: Thirty to forty lymph nodes that are located in the underarm area. Breast cancer cells can travel to the lymph nodes. So, during a modified radical mastectomy, some axillary lymph nodes are removed to test them for the presence of cancer cells.

axillary lymph node dissection: The surgical removal of most of the lymph nodes found in the armpit region.

axillary lymph nodes sampling: The surgical removal of some of the lymph nodes found in the armpit region.

breast reconstruction: The surgical creation of the breast contour, nipple and areola. Performed by a plastic surgeon.

breast self-examination (BSE): The examination of the chest and breast by a woman herself.

chemotherapy: Anti-cancer cytotoxic (cell killing) drugs. Chemotherapy is administered when there is the risk that cancer cells have spread outside of the breast.

clinical breast examination: An examination of the chest, breast and lymph nodes performed by a health provider. The examination usually consists of a visual and a palpation (touch) examination.

ducts: The channels in the breast that carry milk out to the nipple. See invasive or infiltrating breast cancer.

estrogen: A female hormone. See hormone assay test.

hormone assay test: The tumor is tested to see if the cells are receptive to estrogen and progesterone. This procedure is helpful in determining whether the cancer cells are slow or fast growing. It is also helpful when you and your doctors consider tamoxifen (Novadex).

immune system: The body's system to promote healing and to kill viruses, bacteria and cancer cells.

inspection: To examine visually.

invasive or infiltrating breast cancer: Breast cancer that has broken out of the milk ducts and/or lobules and invaded the surrounding breast tissue. Invasive or infiltrating does not imply that the cancer is fast growing or has spread outside of the breast.

lobules: The part of the breast that produces milk. See invasive or infiltrating breast cancer.

lumpectomy: A surgical procedure that removes the cancer and a rim of healthy tissue around the tumor. This breast conservation procedure is usually followed by five to seven weeks of radiation therapy to the breast and chest. A radiation oncologist is a doctor who is a specialist in the treatment of cancer with radiation. A discussion with a radiation oncologist is helpful when deciding whether to have a mastectomy or a lumpectomy.

lymphedema: The chronic swelling of the hand and/or arm. This condition is a possible complication from removing or radiating the lymph nodes under the arm on the side of the mastectomy. Lymphedema can and should be treated. Left untreated, your hand or arm can continue to get larger.

lymph nodes: Small bean-shaped glands found throughout the body that help eliminate bacteria, viruses and cancer cells.

mastectomy: The surgical removal of the breast. A modified radical mastectomy removes the breast and some of the lymph nodes under the arm. A simple mastectomy removes the breast.

metastasis: The spread of breast cancer cells to another organ, such as the lungs, liver, brain or bone.

oncology: The study of cancer.

oncology nurse: A nurse who specializes in the care and recovery of persons with cancer. She is a good resource for information on support groups, breast forms, books and videos.

oncologist: A doctor who specializes in the treatment of cancer, such as a medical oncologist, who specializes in the treatment of cancer with medication; a radiation oncologist, who specializes in the treatment of cancer with radiation therapy; or a surgical oncologist, who specializes in the treatment of cancer with surgery.

pathologist: A doctor who specializes in examining tissue under a microscope and diagnosing disease.

palpation: Examination by touch.

pectoralis major and minor: The major muscles that lie under the breast and over the rib cage.

plastic surgeon: A doctor who specializes in surgically creating a breast contour, nipple and areola.

progesterone: A female hormone. See hormone assay tests.

prosthesis (breast): An artificial breast form.

tamoxifen (Novadex): Medication for breast cancer that reduces the rate of recurrence.

Questions To Ask Your Doctors

QUESTIONS BEFORE SURGERY

◆ What kind of procedure are your recommending?

◆ What are the risks and side effects of the procedure?

◆ Am I a candidate for immediate breast reconstruction?

◆ Am I a candidate for a lumpectomy (a procedure that removes the cancer and preserves the breast)?

◆ What are the advantages and disadvantages of one treatment over another?

◆ How long will I be in the hospital?

◆ How should I expect to look after the operation?

Notes

QUESTIONS REGARDING TAMOXIFEN:

◆ What are the risks and benefits of taking tamoxifen?

◆ How long do I need to take it?

◆ How often do I need to have a pap smear and pelvic examination?

◆ Do I need any other tests on a regular basis if I take tamoxifen?

◆ What are some other possible side effects of tamoxifen?

QUESTIONS REGARDING CHEMOTHERAPY:

◆ What medications do you suggest?

◆ How effective are these drugs in cases similar to mine?

◆ What are the risks and benefits?

◆ How long will I be on chemotherapy?

◆ What can be done to reduce the side effects?

◆ Will I be able to work while on chemotherapy?

◆ How often will I need to see you after treatment ends?

Notes

Questions Regarding Radiation Therapy:

◆ How long will the daily treatments last and how long will I be in the radiation therapy department?

◆ How many weeks will the treatments take?

◆ What are the risks and benefits?

◆ What are the common side effects?

◆ What can be done to reduce the side effects?

◆ How often will I need to see you after treatment ends?

Questions After Your Treatment is Completed:

◆ How often do I need to return for examinations?

◆ How often do I need to have a mammogram?

◆ What other kinds of tests do I need to have, and how often do they need to be done?

Notes

Drain Care Chart

Record the date and the amount of drainage in the appropriate column.

Drain #1

DATE	MORNING	EVENING	TOTAL

Drain #2

DATE	MORNING	EVENING	TOTAL

Resources

*T*he resources included in this guide are selective. They were chosen because they are considered to be the best available.

APPEARANCE

Books

Beauty & Cancer, Dane Doan Noyes and Peggy Mellody, R.N., Taylor Pub. Dallas, Texas, 1992, 163 p. The authors have customized makeup, wardrobe, and other beauty concerns to the specific needs of a woman undergoing chemotherapy, radiation therapy and/or surgery. The guide covers the wearing of scarves, wigs, make-up, clothing, breast forms and makeup. Contact:

> Taylor Publishing
> 1550 South Mockingbird Lane
> Dallas, Texas 75235
> 1-800-275-8188

Feminine Image is a free mail order catalog that features an extensive selection of lingerie and sportswear for the post-breast surgery woman. Beautiful fashions and breast forms from name brand manufacturers and specialty designers are available.

> Feminine Image
> 312 Crosstown Drive, Suite 168
> Peachtree City, Georgia 30269
> 1-800-730-1123

Breast Forms

Amoena Corporation manufactures temporary and permanent breast forms. They manufacture "Affinity," a form that can be worn directly on the body without a bra. For the nearest dealer, contact:

> Amoena Corporation
> 2150 New Market Parkway
> Marietta, Georgia 30067
> 1-800-7-AMOENA (1-800-726-6362)

Coloplast manufactures temporary and permanent breast forms. They manufacture "Discrene," a breast form that can be worn directly on the body without a bra. For the nearest dealer, contact:

> Coloplast, Inc.
> 5610 W. Sligh Avenue, Suite 100-C,
> Tampa, Fl 33634-4468
> 1-800-237-4555

"Softee." The "Softee" is a specially-designed, comfortable camisole with built-in detachable temporary breast forms. Individual inner pockets securely hold the breast form in place, on one or both sides. You can wear the "Softee" home from the hospital and continue wearing it until you get a more permanent form. Contact:

> Ladies First, Inc.
> P.O. Box 4400
> Salem, Oregon 97302
> 1-800-497-8285

Programs

"Look Good. Feel Better." A free workshop for women undergoing treatment for cancer. The workshop covers using turbans, scarves, wigs and make-up. Sponsored by the Cosmetic, Toiletry and Fragrance Association Foundation in partnership with the American Cancer Society and the National Cosmetology Association. Contact:

> 1-800-395-LOOK (1-800-395-5665)

Private Consultation

Peggy Knight International offers private consultation and fitting for wigs, hairpieces, turbans, make-up, bras and breast forms.

> Peggy Knight International
> 32 Ross Common, Box 1499
> Ross, CA 94957
> 1-800-333-8018

BREAST SELF-EXAMINATION

Programs

Mammatech Corporation has developed an effective step-by-step home program to teach breast self-examination. It includes a life-like breast model and a 45 minute videotape. The breast model helps women distinguish a lump from the normal lumpy feeling of the breast. Contact:

> Mammatech Corporation
> 930 Northwest 8th Avenue
> Gainesville, Florida 32601
> 1-800-626-2273

American Cancer Society (ACS). ACS public education programs teach breast self-examination. For services in your area call:

> 1-800-ACS-2345 (1-800-227-2345)

EMOTIONAL RECOVERY

Books

No Less A Women: Ten Women Shatter The Myths About Breast Cancer. Deborah H. Kahane, M.S.W. Prentice-Hall Press, 1990, 279 p. Ten women discuss their personal stories and strategies for coping. Positive and inspiring. Written by a psychotherapist who is a breast cancer survivor. In bookstores.

Spinning Straw Into Gold: Your Emotional Recovery From Breast Cancer. Ronnie Kaye, M.F.C.C. Fireside/Simon & Schuster, Inc., 1991, Paperback. 224 p. Written by a psychotherapist who is a breast cancer survivor. In bookstores.

Invisible Scars. Mimi Greenberg, Ph.D. St. Martin's Press, New York, 1988, 204 p. A down-to-earth helpful, practical guide to coping with the emotional impact of breast cancer. Written by a psychotherapist who is a breast cancer survivor. In bookstores.

Programs

The YWCA Encore Program. This program offers local support groups and exercises classes after mastectomy. Contact:

> YWCA Encore Program
> YWCA National Headquarters
> 726 Broadway
> New York, NY 10003
> 1-212-614-2700

Reach For Recovery Program. This free program is run by local chapters of the American Cancer Society (ACS). Provides one-to-one emotional support and information. Trained volunteers are breast cancer survivors. They can visit you at home or in the hospital, and they can give you a free temporary breast form. For services in your area call:

> 1-800-ACS-2345 (1-800-227-2345)

EXERCISE

Books

Walking Program for People With Cancer. Getting Started. Maryl Winningham, R.N., Ph.D. 1991, 9 p. An easy-to-follow illustrated manual that describes a safe and effective walking program. You can obtain a free copy by contacting:

> Rhythmic Walking
> Suite 1132, James Cancer Hospital
> 300 West Tenth Avenue
> Columbus, Ohio 43210
> 1-614-293-3304

Videos

Beginning Ballet For The Post-Mastectomy Women. Pattie Bryson, breast cancer survivor, nurse, and ballet instructor, demonstrates step-by-step instruction that encourages flexibility and upper-body strengthening. 50 min. Order from:

> First Position Production
> Star Route Box 472
> Sausalito CA 94965
> 1-415-381-9034

Get Up And Go. After Breast Surgery. Exercise program that includes, warm-up, wall and pole exercises, stretching and toning, and meditation. Order by mail or phone:

> Health Tapes, Inc.
> 13320 North End Avenue
> Oak Park, MI 48237
> 1-313-548-2500

Programs

YWCA Encore Program. Water and floor exercises specially developed for women who have had breast cancer surgery. A women can join the group as early as three weeks after surgery. Call your local YWCA or contact the national office:

> YWCA Encore Program
> YWCA National Headquarters
> 726 Broadway
> New York, NY 10003
> 1-212-614-2700

HEALTH INSURANCE

Books

An Almanac of Practical Resources For Cancer Survivors, Charting the Journey. National Coalition for Cancer Survivorship (NCCS). Consumers Union, 1990, 225 p. A comprehensive collection of resources. Includes information and strategies to help with health insurance concerns. Order from:

> NCCS
> 1010 Wayne Avenue, 5th Floor
> Silver Spring, MD 20910
> 1-301-650-8868

Organizations

National Insurance Consumer Organization. An organization formed to educate consumers about their insurance rights, through publication and telephone inquiries. Contact:

> 1-703-549-8050

LYMPHEDEMA

Books & Pamphlets

Recovery In Motion. Linda T. Miller, P.T. 1992, 13 p. An exercise program to assist in the management of upper extremity lymphedema. To order, contact:

> Linda T. Miller, P.T.
> Breast Cancer Physical Therapy Center, Ltd.
> 1905 Spruce Street
> Philadelphia, PA 19103
> 1-215-772-0160

Organization

The National Lymphedema Network (NLN). The NLN provides education regarding the prevention and treatment of lymphedema. Hotline offers support, information and referrals for treatment of lymphedema. Quarterly newsletter. Contact:

> National Lymphedema Network
> 2211 Post Street, Suite 404
> San Francisco, Ca 94115
> 1-800-541-3259

NUTRITION

Books & Pamphlets

Eating Hints: Recipes and Tips For Better Nutrition During Cancer Treatment. 1990, 95 p. This free cookbook-style booklet includes recipes and suggestions for maintaining optimum yet realistic nutrition during treatment. Originally produced by Yale-New Haven Medical Center and reprinted by the NCI. Contact:

> Cancer Information Service
> 1-800-422-6237

Diet, Nutrition and Cancer Prevention: A Guide To Food Choices. 1984, 39 p. This is a free booklet published by the National Institute of Health. It describes what is known about diet, nutrition and cancer prevention. It provides current information about food components (fiber, fat and vitamins) that affect the risk of developing cancer, and suggests ways to use the information, while selecting a variety of food. Contact:

> Cancer Information Service
> 1-800-422-6237

ORGANIZATIONS

American Cancer Society (ACS). A national non-profit organization with local chapters that provides education and patient service programs. "Reach For Recovery" is a program that provides one-to-one emotional support and information by trained volunteers who are breast cancer survivors. "Look Good. Feel Better." is a free workshop for woman under-going treatment for cancer. The workshop covers using turbans, scarves, wigs and make-up. For services in your area call:

> 1-800-ACS-2345 (1-800-227-2345)

Breast Cancer Action. This is an activist and advocacy organization of breast cancer survivors and their supporters, who want to increase the empha-sis on breast cancer in the government, the scientific community, private industry and the media. They have an excellent bi-monthly newsletter. Contact:

> Breast Cancer Action
> 1280 Columbus Ave., Suite 204
> San Francisco, CA 94133
> 1-415-922-8279

National Alliance of Breast Cancer Organizations (NABCO). Provides infor-mation on breast cancer as well as information on regional organizations that offer support to breast cancer survivors. Quarterly newsletter. Contact:

> NABCO
> 1180 Avenue of the Americas, Second floor
> New York, NY 10036
> 1-212-719-0154

Susan G. Komen Breast Cancer Foundation. This is a national organization that supports breast cancer research, education, screening and treatment. Trained volunteers answer a helpline to provide emotional support, information and support group referrals. Contact:

   1-800-IM-AWARE (1-800-462-9273)

The Cancer Information Service (CIS) of the National Cancer Institute (NCI). The NCI is part of the National Institute of Health and is the federal government's principal agency for cancer research and control. The CIS offers free written material and information about treatment, support services, medical facilities, second opinion centers and clinical trials. Trained information specialists answer cancer-related questions:

   1-800-4-CANCER (1-800-422-6237)

The National Coalition For Cancer Survivorship (NCCS). The NCCS is a national coalition of individuals, organizations, and institutions dedicated to survivorship and support of people with cancer and their families. This organization helps locate support groups and resources, serves as an advocate for the rights of cancer survivors, and promotes the study of survivorship. Quarterly newsletter. Contact:

   NCCS
   1010 Wayne Avenue, 5th Floor
   Silver Spring MD, 20910
   1-301-650-8868

Y-Me National Breast Organization For Cancer Information and Support. Y-Me is a non-profit organization providing information, peer support and referral. It also offers information on treatment options, workshops and supports groups. Y-Me has a network of chapters throughout the country that offer local support group meetings. Callers can talk with trained volunteers who are breast cancer survivors. Contact:

> Y-Me
> 18220 Harwood Avenue
> Homewood, IL 60430
> 1-800-221-2141

SEXUALITY

Books & Pamphlets

Sexuality and Cancer: For The Woman Who Has Cancer, and Her Partner 1988, 40 p. This free booklet gives clear, honest information about cancer and sexuality. American Cancer Society publication. Call:

> 1-800-ACS-2345 (1-800-227-2345)

Up Front: Sex And The Post Mastectomy Woman. Linda Dackman. Penguin paperback, 1991, 128 p. Honest, intimate and funny account by a single woman who is a breast cancer survivor in her 30's. In bookstores.

Organizations

American Association of Sex Educators, Counselors, and Therapists (AASECT). A professional organization of trained sex educators, counselors and therapists. For a list of qualified therapists in your state, send a $2.00 check or money order and a self-addressed stamped envelope to:

> AASECT
> 435 North Michigan Avenue, Suite 1717
> Chicago, IL 60611-4067
> 1-312-644-0828

Products

Astroglide. A non-prescription, water-based vaginal lubricant. It is free of scents or flavors. If you would like more information, contact:

> Bio Film, Inc.
> 3121 Scott Street
> Vista, CA 92083
> 1-800-325-5695

Probe. A non-prescription, water-based vaginal lubricant. It is tasteless, odorless, exceptionally slippery and composed primarily of water. If you would like more information, contact:

> Davryan Laboratories, Inc.
> 2623 S.W. Park Place
> Portland, Oregon 97201
> 1-800-637-7623

Replense. A non-prescription vaginal lotion that replenishes vaginal moisture. It is greaseless, non-staining, fragrance free, non-irritating and contains no estrogen. If you would like more information, contact:

> Warner-Lambert Co.
> Parke-Davis
> Morris Plains, NJ 07950
> 1-800-524-2624

TREATMENT

Books

Coping With Chemotherapy. Nancy Bruning. Ballantine Books. New York, 1992, 327 p. A comprehensive overview of the medical, physical and emotional aspects of chemotherapy written by a breast cancer survivor who had chemotherapy. Contains a list of standard drugs and their side effects, and a glossary of terms. In bookstores.

Dr. Susan Love's Breast Book. Susan M. Love, M.D & Kaen Lindsey. Addison-Wesley, 1990, 455 p. Written by a surgeon. This is an easy-to-understand presentation of all aspects of breast cancer from diagnosis to recovery. In bookstores.

If You've Thought About Breast Cancer... Rose Kushner. 1991, 44 pgs. An easy-to-understand pamphlet covering all aspects of breast cancer detection, diagnoses, and treatment. Order from:

> Y-Me
> 18220 Harwood Avenue
> Homewood, IL 60430
> 1-800-221-2141

Radiation Therapy and You: A Guide To Self-Help During Treatment. 1990, 37 p. This is a free pamphlet offered by the National Institute of Health. It contains easy-to-understand information about taking care of yourself during radiation treatment. To order call:

> Cancer Information Service
> 1-800-422-6237

Important Telephone Numbers

Name
Address
Phone

Name
Address
Phone

Name
Address
Phone

Name
Address
Phone

Name
Address
Phone

Name
Address
Phone

Index

Author

Rosalind Dolores Benedet, N.P., M.S.N. is the clinical nurse specialist at the Breast Health Center of California Pacific Medical Center in San Francisco, California. She received her nursing degree and a Master's in Nursing Science at the M.G.H. Institute of Health Professions in Boston, Massachusetts. She is a certified nurse practitioner in women's health. She is a native of San Francisco.

Editor

Edith (Edie) L. Folb, Ph.D. is a professor of Speech and Communication Studies at San Francisco State University. She has taught a variety of courses during her 17 years at SFSU, including intercultural communication, interpersonal communication, oral literature, and women's communicative behavior. She has published extensively on topics ranging from women's language and culture to African American language use to multicultural education. Before coming to SFSU, she taught at UCLA, UCSD, UC Irvine and at the Women's Building in Los Angeles. She has long been an advocate of women's rights in education and health care.

Illustrator

Shannon K. Abbey grew up in Pullman, Washington. She began her formal art training at Western Washington University, studying photography. Just before graduation, she discovered painting and drawing of the human figure. She continued her education at the Academy of Art College in San Francisco, receiving a second Bachelor's degree, this time in illustration. Ms. Abbey lives in San Francisco.

Production Manager

M.J. Coleman, wife, mother and professional, has spent her working career in the creative field, serving as Vice President, Creative Services for Bank of America, heading her own design company, M.J. Coleman Design, and currently representing San Francisco-based Heiney & Craig, Inc., one of the largest annual report and collateral design firms in California.

"After having a bilateral mastectomy and reconstructive surgery last year, I was disappointed with the limited amount of information available for women like me. I wished there had been a book that answered so many of the questions I had before and after my surgery. When asked to assist with *Healing — A Woman's Guide to Recovery After Mastectomy,* I didn't hesitate because I knew there were others like me looking for answers."

Financial Contribution

Dr. Richard Cohen, Cancer Fund of the California Pacific Medical Center in San Francisco, California provided a generous grant that made the printing of this book possible.

Sharron Long was diagnosed with breast cancer the same year her sister Judy Hill died of the disease. Her association with the author is the result of her desire to make a contribution to the breast cancer community in her sister's name; hence, the dedication of this book. It is her hope that this will be a "working" memorial to her sister in that it will help breast cancer patients everywhere deal with their diagnosis and begin their healing process.

Order Form

*P*lease send me additional copies of "Healing – A Woman's Guide To Recovery After Mastectomy"

NAME: _____

COMPANY: _____

ADDRESS: _____

CITY/STATE/ZIP: _____

TELEPHONE: _____

To order

Send $10.00 plus shipping ($1.00 for the first book, $.25 for each additional book; for 2-day rush order, $3.00 for one book, $.25 for each additional book). California residents add 85¢ sales tax per book. All orders must be prepaid.

Discount available for orders of 10 or more. For information on volume orders call 415-281-3380.

Please send me _____ copy(ies) $ _____

Regular Shipping $1.00 $ _____

Please Rush the Shipping $3.00 $ _____

California Sales Tax (85¢ per book) $ _____

Total: $ _____

Make Check Payable to: R. Benedet Publishing
                            220 Montgomery Street, Penthouse #2
                            San Francisco, California 94104